AMPICILLIN

The Best Guide To Treat Bacterial, Pneumonia, and Other Infections of The Respiratory Tract.

DR

ETHAN

OLIVER

INTRODUCTION

Antibiotics are drugs that kill or inhibit the development of bacteria. They are prescribed by physicians to treat bacterial infections. They accomplish this by eliminating bacteria and preventing their multiplication.

They include a variety of potent medications used to treat bacterial diseases.

Antibiotics are potent medications that can save lives when used properly to treat certain infections. They either prevent the reproduction of bacteria or eliminate them.

Typically, the immune system can eliminate microorganisms before they multiply and cause symptoms. White blood cells (WBCs) attack harmful pathogens; even in the presence of symptoms, the immune system is typically able to combat the infection.

Occasionally, however, there are too many harmful microbes for the immune system to eliminate. Antibiotics are beneficial in this circumstance.

Penicillin was the first antibiotic discovered. Antibiotics based on penicillin, such as ampicillin, and amoxicillin, are still available and have been used for many years to treat a variety of infections.

Why is it crucial to take antibiotics whenever they are prescribed?

Antibiotics should only be utilized when necessary, according to the recommendations of experts. This is done to guarantee that the bacteria are eradicated and that they are unable to reproduce or spread to other areas of the body.

In addition, the usage of antibiotics is sometimes linked to the development of adverse effects and antibiotic resistance.

CHAPTER 1

WHAT'S AMPICILLIN?

Ampicillin is an antibiotic that is used to treat infections caused by germs in the middle ear, sinuses, stomach, intestines, kidney, and bladder. It is also used to treat serious infections like meningitis, endocarditis, and gonorrhea that is not complex.

Ampicillin is a type of drug called penicillin, which is used to treat infections caused by bacteria. Amoxicillin (Amoxil), ticarcillin (Ticar), and piperacillin (Pipracil), a few others are also in this class. Each of these medicines works similarly.

Inform your doctor if you are pregnant or intend to become pregnant while taking this medication. It is recommended to avoid taking Ampicillin if –

You are allergic to all penicillin-based antibiotics.

You are taking antibiotics containing tetracycline or mononucleosides.

You have recently received a vaccination or will soon receive a vaccination.

Ampicillin has a lower toxicity compared to other antibiotics. Side effects are uncommon and infrequent. They include vertigo, vomiting, a high eosinophil count, skin rashes, tongue swelling, and diarrhea. Serious but uncommon adverse reactions include persistent sore throat, dark urine, jaundice, abdominal pain, easy bruising or bleeding, persistent sore pharynx, and fever.

The prescribed dosage of this medication depends on your age, kidney function, and the variety of bacteria causing the infection. It is typically consumed four times a day, every six hours, or as directed by a physician. Inappropriate or excessive use of this medication will diminish its efficacy.

Even if you feel better, you must finish the entire prescription.

Take at equal intervals around the clock, preferably on an empty stomach with a full glass of water (1 hour before or 2 hours after meals).

Maintain adequate hydration (two to three liters (L) of fluids per day, unless otherwise instructed). You may experience vertigo or vomiting (small frequent meals, sucking lozenges, frequent mouth care, or chewing gum may be beneficial).

Ampicillin can be taken by mouth (pills, syrup, dispersible tablets, capsules, oral drops, dry syrup, suspension), or it can be given as an injection.

CHAPTER 2

COMMON USES OF AMPICILLIN

What is the intended use?

- **Infection of the Abdomen**

In the treatment of intra-abdominal infections, ampicillin is utilized. It is a general term that encompasses a variety of infections of the abdominal organs. It contains:

Peritonitis (inflammation and infection of the membrane lining the abdominal wall, which protects the organs within the abdomen)

Diverticulitis (is an inflammation of the diverticula, which are tiny pouches in the intestine).

Cholecystitis (gallbladder inflammation)

Cholangitis (bile duct system inflammation)

Pancreatitis (pancreatic inflammation)

- **For The Disease Shigellosis**

Shigellosis is an intestinal infection brought on by the bacterium Shigella. The symptoms include bloody diarrhea, severe abdominal pain, and fever, among others. For the treatment of Shigella infections, ampicillin is utilized.

- **Typhoid Fever**

Salmonella typhi causes typhoid fever, which is a bacterial infection. It is transmitted via contaminated food and water. Symptoms may include a high fever, headache, abdominal pain, vomiting, loose feces, and weakness, among others. Ampicillin is utilized to treat typhoid fever.

- **Chronic pharyngitis**

Pharyngitis, also known as sore throat, is an infection of the throat and tonsils (tissue nodules located at the back of the esophagus). Symptoms may include trouble swallowing, a dry or itchy larynx, throat pain, headache, and body aches, among others. Ampicillin is utilized to treat pharyngitis

- **Urinary Tract Infection**

Urinary Tract Infection refers to any infection of the urinary system. It may impact the kidneys, urinary bladder, ureter, or urethra. Symptoms may include an increased need to urinate, a burning sensation during urination, the presence of blood in the urine, back discomfort, fever, etc. The antibiotic ampicillin is used to treat urinary tract infections.

- **Gastroenteritis**

The infection of the stomach and intestines known as gastroenteritis is also known as the stomach virus. The symptoms include diarrhea, vomiting, fever, and nausea. For the treatment of gastroenteritis, ampicillin is utilized.

- **Bronchopulmonary infection**

Pneumonia is an infection of the lungs that can affect one or both lungs. Possible causes include bacteria, viruses, and fungi. Ampicillin is utilized in the treatment of bacterial pneumonia.

- **Serious Bronchitis**

Bronchitis is the inflammation of the tubes that carry oxygen to and from the lungs. Coughing and shortness of breath are typical symptoms. The antibiotic ampicillin is used to treat bronchitis caused by bacteria.

- **Chronic sinusitis**

Sinuses are the hollow spaces behind the forehead, nostrils, cheeks, and between the eyes. Sinusitis is an inflammation of the sinuses' adjacent tissues. The symptoms include a stuffy nose, a headache, and discomfort or pressure behind the eyes, the nose, the cheeks, or the forehead. The antibiotic ampicillin is used to treat bacterial sinusitis.

- **Meningitis Caused By Bacteria**

Meningitis is an infection that causes swelling of the membranes that encircle the brain and spinal cord. The antibiotic ampicillin is used to treat bacterial meningitis.

- **Gonorrhea**

Gonorrhea is a sexually transmitted illness (STI) that is caused by the Neisseria gonorrhea bacteria. It spreads through sexual contact that is not protected. Ampicillin is a drug that is used to treat gonorrhea.

- **Bacterial Septicaemia**

Septicaemia, also called sepsis, is a blood illness caused by bacteria. Some of the symptoms are a fast heartbeat, trouble breathing, tiredness or weakness, diarrhea, sickness or vomiting, etc. Ampicillin is used to treat septicemia, which is caused by bacteria.

CHAPTER 3

AMPICILLIN SIDE EFFECTS

Possible adverse reactions to this medication include the following:

- Diarrhea
- Red, itchy rash
- Injection Site Pain
- Chills and a fever
- Vomiting
- Sensitivity to Allergens
- Anemia

Concerns

Frequently Asked Questions;

Action begins

It is unknown how long Ampicillin takes to take effect.

The duration of the influence

Ampicillin might stay in your system for up to 9 hours after being taken orally. It is unknown how long this medication stays in your system following an intravenous infusion.

Is it safe to drink alcohol?

Alcohol interaction is unknown. It is best to see your doctor before using this product.

Is it creating a habit?

Ampicillin has not been associated with any habit-forming properties.

Use while pregnant?

Ampicillin is safe to use to treat bacterial illnesses during pregnancy. Use this medicine only as directed by your doctor.

Use while a baby is nursing?

Very little ampicillin is found in breast milk. If you are nursing, your baby might have diarrhea from time to time. So, before you take this medicine, you should talk to your doctor.

When not to use it?

<u>Allergic reactions</u>

If you are allergic to ampicillin, it is not a good idea to use it. See a doctor right away if you have signs like a rash, itching, or swelling (especially in the face, tongue, or throat), severe dizziness, trouble breathing, etc.

CHAPTER 4

DOSAGE OF AMPICILLIN
How to use ampicillin

This is how much ampicillin oral pill to take. This list may not have all of the possible doses and drug forms. How much you should take, what form it comes in, and how often you take it will depend on:

1. How old you are and what is being treated

2. How bad your situation is and what other health problems you have you have to see how the first dose makes you feel.
3. The doses listed below are for the most common diseases that this drug is used to treat.

This list might not have all of the reasons why your doctor can give you this drug. Talk to your doctor if you have any questions about your medicine.

Infections Of The Genitourinary Tract or Gonorrhea Dosage

Dosage for adults (18–64 years)

For infections of the **genitourinary tract** other than gonorrhea:

The standard dosage is 500 mg four times daily.

Infections that are severe or chronic may require higher dosages.

Regarding **gonorrhea**:

The typical dosage is 3.5 grams administered once, along with 1 gram of probenecid.

Children weighing more than 20 kg (child dosage)

Other than gonorrhea, for genitourinary tract infections:

Four times a day, 500 milligrams is the typical dosage.

Dosage for Children weighing less than 20 kg.

For infections of the genitourinary system:

The standard dosage is 100 mg/kg per day, divided and separated into four equal doses.

Dosage for the elderly (65 and older)

The kidneys of elderly individuals may not function as well as they once did. This can slow the body's ability to metabolize drugs. As a consequence, more drug remains in the body for a longer period. This increases the likelihood of side effects.

Your physician may prescribe a reduced dose or a different schedule. This can prevent excessive levels of this substance from accumulating in the body.

Dosage for upper respiratory infections

Dosage for adults (18–64 years)

The normal daily dosage is four times 250 mg.

Dosage for Children(0 to 17 years old and weighing more than 20 kg).

The normal daily dosage is four times 250 mg.

<u>Child dosage (0–17-year-olds weighing less than 20 kg).</u>

The typical dosage is 50 mg/kg per day, administered in three to four equally divided and spaced doses.

<u>Dosage for the elderly (65 and older)</u>

The kidneys of elderly individuals may not function as well as they once did. This can slow the body's ability to metabolize drugs. As a consequence, more drug remains in the body for a longer period. This increases the likelihood of side effects.

Your physician may prescribe a reduced dose or a different schedule. This can prevent excessive levels of this substance from accumulating in the body.

Gastrointestinal Tract Infection Dosage

<u>Dosage for adults (18–64 years)</u>

The standard dosage is 500 mg four times daily.

The standard dosage is 500 mg four times daily.

<u>Pediatric dosage (for Children weighing more than 20 kg).</u>

The standard dosage Is 500 mg four times daily.

Dosage for Children weighing 20 kg or less.

The typical daily dosage is 100 mg/kg divided into four evenly spaced doses.

Dosage for the elderly (aged 65 and up)

Elderly individuals' kidneys may not function as effectively as they once did. This can result in a slower metabolism of pharmaceuticals. Consequently, more of a drug remains in the body for a prolonged duration. This increases the chance of adverse effects.

Your physician may begin you on a reduced dose or a different schedule. This can prevent excessive accumulation of this drug in your body.

Meningitis Dosage

Dosage for adults (ages 18–64)

The right dose for you will be decided by your doctor.

Dosage for children (0–17 years old)

The right dose for your child will be decided by the doctor.

Dosage for seniors (ages 65 and up)

People who are getting older may not have kidneys that work as well as they used to. This can make your body take longer to break down drugs. Because of this, your body keeps more of a drug for a longer time. This makes it more likely that you will feel bad.

Your doctor may give you a lower dose or a different plan to follow at first. This can help keep you from getting too much of this drug in your body.

CHAPTER 5

AMPICILLIN INTERACTIONS

Taking ampicillin with certain other medications increases the likelihood of experiencing side effects from ampicillin. This is because the ampicillin concentration in your body may increase. Examples of such medications include:

The drug **Probenecid**

Combining this medication with ampicillin may increase side effects. These symptoms may include vomiting, nausea, and diarrhea.

The drug **allopurinol**

When taken with ampicillin, this medication increases the risk of skin rash.

Interactions that can reduce the efficacy of your medications

When ampicillin effectiveness declines: When combined with certain antibiotics, ampicillin may be less effective in treating your condition. This is because these antibiotics inhibit bacterial proliferation, whereas ampicillin requires bacteria to multiply to kill them. Examples of such medications include:

Tetracyclines, macrolides, sulfamides, and chloramphenicol

When other medications are ineffective: When certain pharmaceuticals are combined with ampicillin, their effectiveness may be diminished. This is because the concentration of these medications in your body may decrease. Several examples include:

Birth control tablets (oral contraceptives)

Your physician may prescribe a different method of contraception.

CHAPTER 6

General Guidelines

Ampicillin oral formulations: Take 1 hour before or 2 hours after meals. Do not exceed or decrease the prescribed dosage.

Even if you feel improved after a few doses, you must finish the entire course of medication. If you stop taking the medication, your risk of infection may increase. In addition, Ampicillin may lose its efficacy against infections.

Avoid recommending Ampicillin to others, even if their condition seems similar to yours.

Before using syrup, suspension, or drops, shake the bottle vigorously. Use a measuring utensil or dropper to administer Ampicillin exactly as prescribed by your doctor.

Dry syrup: Put the mixture back together by adding the right amount of clean water and shaking it well. Use a measuring spoon or dropper to get the right amount.

Dispersible Tablet: Before taking this medicine, mix it with a teaspoon of water or a glass of water.

Injection: A qualified healthcare worker in a clinic or hospital gives an ampicillin injection.

Alcoholic Interaction

Alcohol interaction is unknown. Before consumption, it is advised to consult with a physician.

CHAPTER 7

Warnings For Individuals With Specific Medical Conditions

This medication may induce a false positive result in urine tests for glucose (sugar) in diabetic patients. This means that the test may falsely indicate that you have glucose in your urine. Ask your physician if this drug is safe for you to take.

For individuals with kidney issues: If you have kidney issues or a history of kidney disease, you may not be able to eliminate this drug from your body effectively. This may increase the drug's concentration in the body, resulting in more adverse effects.

For nursing mothers: Ampicillin may transfer into breast milk and cause adverse effects in a nursing infant. Consult your physician if you are breastfeeding your child. You may have to choose between stopping breastfeeding and stopping this medication.

The kidneys of older individuals may not function as well as they once did. This can slow the body's ability to metabolize drugs. As a consequence, more drug remains in the body for a longer period. This increases the likelihood of side effects.

Newborns and infants should take the lowest feasible dose of this medication. The reason for this is that their kidneys are not completely developed. It could take longer for this substance to leave their system. This means that it may have more adverse effects.

Made in United States
Troutdale, OR
03/11/2024

18364853R00030